How To Rock
At the Elimination Diet

By Erin Germaine

This guidebook has been crafted for you with care by Erin Germaine, Certified Holistic Nutritionist, Wellness Coach, and lover of all foods. After three years of researching, here is the plan to get you to move past those funks, and fight through the fog to a better version of yourself.

Don't forget, you totally rock!

Preface

As frustrating as what you're going through right now might be, I'm excited to say that everything is going to be okay! How do I know this? Because you - like me and so many others - might just have a food sensitivity or allergy. If you aren't sure what is causing your symptoms, this guide was created for you!

I believe in the power of self. Self is able to hold it together, and carry on. I like to think that we were each gifted a set of skills to help ourselves through even the most difficult obstacles. Would it be safe for me to say that you have been struggling with your mood swings, exhaustion, aches, and itches for quite some time? Taking it like a champ does you no good when you're totally wiped and have no explanation as to why!

Are you suffering from relentless brain fog, one that doesn't seem to dissipate no matter how many cups of coffee or espresso? Perhaps finding yourself trudging along with achy joints and muscles - and you know it's not because you just hit the gym?

The constant ups and downs occurring inside you are sort of depressing. But that's a strong word, so perhaps it's *safer* to say that your hair-pulling uncertainty has left you feeling *funky* - and not in a good way!

One time, I was out in public when I noticed that lots of people were looking at me. I was totally flattered, thinking it was the new top I was wearing! I was so embarrassed later when I got back to my car and noticed all of the "Hollywood-attention" was in fact due to the huge red welt (which was the size of my thumb) across my chest! This condition is called dermography, when the skin welts up from very little stimuli (it is interesting as much as it is annoying).

Well, three years ago, I decided that *something* has got to give! I have assembled this guide to help you visualize and attain your goals of a happier, more healthy life. Backed by tons of scientific research (I love me an expert opinion!), I have included a shopping list with menu ideas and recipes to help spark creativity in your kitchen. Your food options will be limited temporarily.

This is *your* guide to completing the Clean Fit Wellness Elimination Diet, a dietary program designed to clean your body of foods and chemicals that you may have an unknown sensitivity. The main idea behind this diet is that specific modifications allow your body's detoxification machinery to recover and begin to function efficiently again.

Certain dietary changes will help the body to *naturally* eliminate toxins that may have accumulated over time from certain lifestyle choices (foods, beverages, drugs, alcohol, cigarette smoke) and other environmental exposures - including additives and chemicals. I always recommend nutrition counseling to help you start with some solid information and accountability. An added benefit: The elimination of toxins reduces inflammation throughout the body resulting in a loss of up to 5 pounds in the first week!

Food Allergy and Intolerance 101

Food intolerance - which is also known as non-immunoglobulin E (non-IgE) around all the doctors - is a food hypersensitivity. A non-allergic food hypersensitivity is simply your body having difficulty digesting certain trigger foods. Non-allergenic foods will *not* trigger the army of white blood cells defending its immune system, which means there is no *histamine* response. But there is a response!

Foods that are most commonly associated with food intolerance include dairy products, grains that contain gluten, and foods that cause intestinal gas buildup, such as beans and cabbage. Here are some symptoms of a food intolerance:

- Gas, cramps, or bloating
- **Heartburn**
- **Headaches**
- Irritability or nervousness

Let's take a closer look at the differences between food allergies, and food sensitivities.

FOOD ALLERGY	FOOD SENSITIVITY

Usually comes on suddenly	Usually comes on gradually
Small amount of food can trigger	May only happen when you eat a lot of that food
Happens every time you eat the food	May only happen if you eat the food often
Can be life-threatening	Is not life-threatening

With a true food allergy, your body's natural defenses will <u>overreact</u> to the exposure to a particular substance, treating it as an invader and sending out chemicals to defend against it.

The symptoms of a histamine (allergic) reaction are:

- Rash, hives, or itchy skin
- Shortness of breath
- Chest pain

The differences are extreme, and allergic reactions should be taken very seriously. However, food sensitivities can dull your daily experiences and should also be handled with seriousness.

I understand how frustrating and isolating the experiences are when you're out with friends and suddenly you get symptoms from something you ate, maybe even hours after you ate it. Or, more frustrating, the moments of panic before a first dinner date because you aren't sure if something on the menu will trigger your ugly friend, "The Rash."

I can always tell when I've eaten something that didn't agree with me because I get "The Fog!" I spend the next day chugging lemon water to chase away the junk from the previous day. And what's worse, is that I anticipate it coming after certain snacks, meals, or drinks. Not fun guys!

You are not alone in your feelings of discomfort. Food sensitivities and allergies have become a common struggle people across America are facing; this is mainly caused by the unnatural chemicals and additives that we are exposed to when buy foods in our own towns.

With the Elimination Diet, you will be able to discover what it is that is causing your symptoms, and in most cases, you will be able to reverse the sensitivity. And you're going to rock at it! I've provided a simple calendar to follow, and have laid out some of the best recipes to use along the way.

If you have any of these symptoms, the Elimination Diet can significantly improve your quality of life:

- Tingling or itching in the mouth
- Hives, itching or eczema
- Swelling of the lips, face, tongue and throat or other parts of the body
- Wheezing, nasal congestion or trouble breathing
- Abdominal pain, diarrhea, nausea or vomiting
- Achy joints or muscles
- Dizziness, lightheadedness or fainting
- Brain fog
- Low ability to focus
- Nausea
- Stomach pain
- **Diarrhea**
- **Vomiting**

This list may be slightly larger, but if you're encountering any or several of these symptoms you're in rough shape to face your daily tasks. Let's get you feeling like the badass that you are. Are you with me?

Beginning Your Journey

For a total of 112 days, you are going to have to pay *very* close attention to the messages your body is sending. Write it down, keep an online diary - make it fun! It sounds like a long time, but once you start feeling better you'll run with this.

Others who have completed the Elimination Diet have documented powerful changes. Many have shared an increased energy, mental alertness, a decrease in muscle or joint pain and a general sense of improved well-being. While this is most common, there is no "typical" or "normal" response.

Keep in mind that your initial response to ANY new diet is highly variable from someone else's, and this diet is no exception! Why, might you ask? Well, the different responses can be linked to physiological, mental and biochemical differences among individuals, also the degree of exposure to, and type of "toxin"...other lifestyle factors. Keep track of it all!

When you're grocery shopping and out at your favorite restaurant, do yourself a favor and make sure to read all labels carefully and ask lots of questions. You want to find any of those hidden allergens before your stomach does.

Eat a wide variety of foods and do not try to restrict your calorie intake. It is important to note that there are no magical answers here, it's just you, your body, and your food (kind of dreamy, huh?). This is your journey of self-exploration and discovery.

It is likely your first week won't be smooth sailing - so mentally prepare for that. Yoga, meditation, a long walk outside. The initial reaction as your body adjusts to a different dietary program could give you symptoms like, itchiness, sweatiness, and restlessness. Not to worry, these symptoms rarely last for more than a few days.

What to expect your first week as your body releases toxins:

- changes in sleep patterns

- lightheadedness
- headaches
- joint or muscle stiffness
- changes in gastrointestinal function

Useful Tips to Use Along the Way!

- The first 2 to 3 days are the hardest. Make it a little easier for yourself by going shopping before you begin to get all of the foods you are allowed to have.
- Plan your meals each week! Don't jump into a brand new week of a brand new you without a clue how you're going to do it! Tip: Make a lot of rice.
- Go for simplicity. Cook and eat simple. Make a pot of chicken-vegetable-rice soup. Make a large salad. Cook extra chicken. Have prepared food on hand so you can grab something quickly.
- Eat your meals regularly. The same time every day.

- You may also want to keep snacks packed to keep your blood sugar stable. Bring your snacks with you so you're not tempted to indulge while you're out - guilty!
- It may be helpful to cook extra chicken, sweet potatoes, rice, beans, etc. that can be reheated for snacking or another meal.
- Avoid any foods that you already know or believe you may be sensitive to, even if they are on the "allowed" list.
- Try to eat at least three servings of fresh vegetables each day. Include at least one serving of dark green or orange vegetables (carrot, broccoli, winter squash) and one raw vegetable each day. You'll want to vary your selections to keep yourself excited and motivated.
- Buy organic produce when possible. Opt for fresh foods whenever you can, and if possible, choose organically grown fruits and vegetables to eliminate pesticide and chemical residue consumption. (Oh, and Always wash fruits and vegetables thoroughly.)
- If you are a vegetarian, eliminate the meat and fish and consume more beans and rice, quinoa, amaranth, teff, millet and buckwheat.
- If you're a stone-cold coffee machine, or heavy on any other caffeine beverages, it'd be better to slowly reduce your caffeine intake rather than abruptly stop it. Caffeine headaches are intense!

- Read oil labels (all labels!) and use only those that have been "cold pressed".
- If you opt for animal protein, look for free-range or organically raised chicken, turkey or lamb. Always trim the visible fat and cook by broiling, baking, stewing, grilling or stir-frying. Cold-water fish (salmon, mackerel, and halibut) is another excellent source of protein and the omega-3 essential fatty acids, which are important nutrients in this diet.
- Get used to using leftovers for the next day or part of a meal (leftover broiled salmon and broccoli from dinner as part of a large salad for lunch the next day). Huge money and time saver!
- Remember to drink the recommended amount (at least two quarts) of plain, filtered water each day.
- Any intense exercise programs can be reduced during some or the entire program to allow the body to heal more effectively. Adequate rest and stress reduction are also important to the success of this program.
- Always remember: You Rock!

The Elimination Diet Calendar

For the first part of each phase, cut the listed foods out of your diet. Then
add each food back, one at a time, for just three days to see if you have any
symptoms (use your Food Journal religiously).

Phase 1

Day 1-21	DAIRY	GLUTEN	SOY	EGGS
Day 22-24	DAIRY			
Day 25-27	DAIRY	GLUTEN		
Day 30-32	DAIRY	GLUTEN	SOY	
Day 33-35	DAIRY	GLUTEN	SOY	EGGS

Phase 2

Day 36-58	PEANUTS	SHELLFISH	CORN
Day 59-61	PEANUTS		
Day 62-64	PEANUTS	SHELLFISH	
Day 65-67	PEANUTS	SHELLFISH	CORN

Phase 3

DAY 68-90	TREE NUTS	FISH
Day 91-93	TREE NUTS	
Day 94-96	TREE NUTS	FISH

Phase 4

Day 97-103	PRESERVATIVES	ARTIFICIAL SUGARS	ARTIFICIAL DYES
Day 104-106	PRESERVATIVES		
Day 107-109	PRESERVATIVES	ARTIFICIAL SUGARS	
Day 110-112	PRESERVATIVES	ARTIFICIAL SUGARS	ARTIFICIAL DYES

The whole Picture

POSSIBLE PROBLEMS: Most people feel better and better each day during the allergy elimination diet. However, if you are used to using caffeine, you may get withdrawal symptoms the first few days which may include: headaches, fatigue irritability, malaise, or increased hunger. If you find your energy lagging, you may need to eat frequently to keep your blood sugar levels (thinking, energy) level. Be sure to drink plenty of water!

TESTING INDIVIDUAL FOODS: Once you've completed three weeks you can begin to add foods back into your diet. Keep a food journal of all foods eaten and symptoms. Add foods one at a time, one every two days. Eat the test food at least twice a day and in a fairly large amount. Often an offending food will provoke symptoms quickly (within in 10 minutes to 12 hours). Signs to look for include: headache, itching, bloating, nausea, dizziness, fatigue, diarrhea, indigestion, anal itching, sleepy 30 minutes after a meal, flushing, rapid heartbeat. If you're still unsure, take the food back out of your diet for at least one week and try it again. Be sure to test foods in a pure form: for example test milk or cheese or wheat, but not macaroni and cheese that contains milk, cheese and wheat!

THE RESULTS: Avoiding the symptom-provoking foods and taking supportive supplements to restore gut integrity (pro/pre biotics) can help most food allergies/sensitivities resolve within 4 to 6 months. This means that in most cases you will be able to again eat foods that formerly bothered you! In some cases, you will find that the sensitivity doesn't go away. In this case you will have to either wait longer for the symptoms to resolve, or it may be a "fixed" allergy that will be lifelong. You can get tested for this.

AFTER THE TESTING: If you find that you have allergies to many foods, you may want to explore a 4-day food rotation diet. Anytime you change your diet significantly, you may experience the symptoms of fatigue, headache or muscle aches for a few days. That's okay, your body needs this time as it "withdraws" from the foods you eat on a daily basis. Your body may crave some foods it is used to consuming. Always be patient your body! Those symptoms generally don't last long, and most people feel much better over the next couple of weeks.

Foods to Include in Your Diet

Fruits: whole fruits, unsweetened, frozen or water-packed, canned fruits and diluted juices.

Dairy substitutes: rice milk

Non-gluten grains and starch: rice (all types), millet, quinoa, amaranth, teff , tapioca, buckwheat, potato flour.

Animal protein: fresh or water-packed canned fish, wild game, lamb, duck, organic chicken and turkey

IF YOU ARE A VEGETARIAN: split peas, lentils and legumes If you are not a vegetarian, do not include these foods.

Nuts and seeds: Coconut, pine nuts, flax seeds

Vegetables: all raw, steamed, sautéed, juiced or roasted vegetables

Oils: cold-pressed olive, ghee

Drinks: filtered or distilled water, decaffeinated herbal teas, seltzer or mineral water

Sweeteners: Use Sparingly: brown rice syrup, agave nectar, stevia, fruit sweetener, blackstrap molasses

Condiments: vinegar, all spices, including salt, pepper, basil, carob, cinnamon, cumin, dill, garlic, ginger, mustard, oregano, parsley, rosemary, tarragon, thyme, turmeric

These May Be Hiding, So Beware!!

- Corn starch in baking powder and any processed foods
- Corn syrup in beverages and processed foods
- Vinegar in ketchup, mayonnaise and mustard is usually from wheat or corn
- Breads advertised as gluten-free which contain oats, spelt, kamut, rye
- Many amaranth and millet flake cereals have oats or corn
- Many canned tunas contain textured vegetable protein which is from soy
- Look for low-salt versions which tend to be pure tuna, with no fillers

Shopping List
Read labels carefully

Fruits	Animal Protein	Dairy Substitutes
Apples, Applesauce, Apricots, Bananas, Blackberries, Blueberries, Cantaloupe, Cherries, Coconut, Figs, Grapefruit, Huckleberries, Kiwi, Kumquat, Lemons, Limes	Free-range Chicken, Turkey, Duck, Fresh Ocean Fish (Pacific Salmon, Halibut, Haddock, Cod, Sole, Pollock, Tuna, Mahi-mahi) Lamb Water-packed Canned Tuna	Almond Milk, Rice Milk, Coconut Milk, Oat Milk **Beans: If you are vegetarian, include these foods. If you are eating animal foods, eliminate these foods.**

Loganberries, Mangos, Melons, Mulberries, Nectarines, Papayas, Peaches, Pears, Prunes, Raspberries, Strawberries *Can all be consumed raw or juiced

Vegetables

Artichoke, Asparagus, Avocado, Bamboo Shoots Beets and Beet Tops, Bok Choy, Broccoflower, Broccoli, Brussels Sprouts Cabbage, *Bell Peppers*, Carrots, Cauliflower, Celery, Chives, Cucumber, Dandelion Greens, *Eggplant*, Endive, Kale, Kohlrabi, Leeks, Lettuce – or green leaf and Chinese, Mushroom, Okra, Onions, Pak-Choi Parsley, Potato, Red Leaf Chicory, Sea Vegetables – Seaweed, Kelp, Snow Peas, Spinach, Squash, Sweet Potatoes and Yams, Swiss Chard, Tomatoes, Watercress, Zucchini

(watch for added protein from soy), Wild game

Oils

Ghee, Flax, Olive, Coconut

Herbs, Spices & Extracts

Basil, Black Pepper, Cinnamon, Cumin, Dandelion, Dill, Dry Mustard, Garlic, Ginger, Nutmeg, Oregano, Parsley, Rosemary Salt-free Herbal Blends Sea Salt, Tarragon, Thyme, Turmeric, Pure Vanilla Extract

Breads & Baking

Arrowroot, Baking Soda, Glut free Breads, Flours: rice, teff, quinoa, millet, tapioca, amaranth, potato, Mochi Rice Bran, Rice Flour Pancake Mix, Rice Tortillas

Non-Gluten Grains

Amaranth, Millet, Quinoa, Rice – brown, white, wild, Teff, Buckwheat, Rice Crackers

Cereals & Pasta

Cream of Rice, Puffed Rice, Puffed Millet, Quinoa Flakes, Rice Pasta, 100 % Buckwheat Noodles, Rice Crackers/Rice Cakes

All beans except soy Lentils - brown, green, red Split peas *Can be dried or canned.*

Nuts

Coconut

Vinegars

Apple cider, Balsamic, Red Wine, Rice, Tarragon Ume Plum

Sweeteners

Fruit sweetener (100 % juice concentrate), Agave Nectar, Molasses, Rice Syrup, Stevia

Condiments

Mustard (made with apple cider vinegar)

Beverages

Herbal Tea (non-caffeinated), Mineral Water, Pure Unsweetened Fruit or Vegetable Juices, Spring Water

*Can all be consumed *Raw, juiced steamed, sautéed or baked. If you have arthritis, avoid nightshades (in italics).*		

Menu Ideas

Breakfast

Feel free to add protein powder drinks, leftover chicken, fish, etc., to your breakfast menu.

- ▢ Cooked whole grain (oatmeal, cream of brown rice, buckwheat, teff, millet or quinoa) served with fresh or frozen fruit. Can add a bit of coconut, ghee, sweetener and/or cinnamon. To boost protein, have rice protein powder drink.
- ▢ Home-fried potatoes: Cut onions, peppers, broccoli, mushrooms and other vegetables of your choice into small pieces and sauté in olive

oil or ghee. Cut pre-baked potatoes into cubes and add to vegetables. Add salt/pepper/herbs/spices

- "Fried" rice: Use recipe above. Add rice instead of potatoes
- Toasted rice or lentil flax bread with coconut oil or ghee, 100 % fruit jam or apple or pear butter, fresh fruit, and herbal tea
- Fruit smoothie: Blend rice milk with fruit. Possible choices: berries, bananas, pears, pineapple, mango, papaya, etc. Add flax seeds or psyllium seeds as desired. Add fish oil as desired. Drink on its own or as part of a breakfast
- Rice pancakes topped with apple butter or applesauce or sautéed apples
- Cold rice or amaranth or other gluten-free cereal (read label carefully) with fresh fruit (bananas, berries, pears, apples, etc) and rice milk
- Sweet potato delight, half a cantaloupe filled with blueberries or half a papaya with lime juice
- Mochi rice waffles, topped with sautéed apples and fruit smoothie with rice protein powder
- Breakfast rice pudding, rice milk, berries

Lunch or Dinner

- Large salad with grilled chicken or fish. Serve with non-gluten containing bread or baked potato or winter squash or boiled new potatoes
- Broiled salmon plus steamed or oven-roasted vegetables with cooked millet or baked potato or sweet potato or quinoa salad. Can also add a salad with vinaigrette dressing
- Asparagus soup (or other soup), cabbage salad, rice cakes with ghee, fresh fruit
- Broiled lamb chop, green rice, cooked vegetables, fruity spinach salad
- Fruit salad with coconut/or pine nuts. Serve with protein and rice crackers
- Broiled or poached halibut, baked winter squash sprinkled with cinnamon and ghee, mixed green salad with vinaigrette dressing, mocha rice squares and fruit for dessert
- Brown rice and grilled chicken, steamed greens, baked potato or sweet potato
- Halibut salad: Mixed greens of your choice, leftover halibut cut into chunks, vinaigrette dressing. Serve with baked potato with ghee

- Chicken breast sprinkled with garlic powder and tarragon, steamed asparagus or broccoli, brown or wild rice or kasha, ghee or olive oil
- Quinoa with chicken-vegetable soup or vegetable soup
- Quinoa salad with leftover chicken or fish
- Chicken salad: leftover chicken, mixed greens, guacamole, millet with pine nuts
- Fresh tuna steak topped with herbs and broiled, rice pasta with olive oil and mock pesto, steamed kale or collard greens tossed with olive oil and garlic and vinegar, mixed green salad with vinaigrette dressing. Fruit for dessert
- Tuna salad: Canned tuna mixed with vinaigrette or eggless mayonnaise, baking powder biscuits, fresh fruit
- Roast turkey breast or broiled turkey burger, brown or wild rice, steamed vegetable, salad with vinaigrette. Baked apple or poached pear
- Turkey salad: leftover turkey breast, mixed greens, other fresh vegetables, lemon or oil and vinegar, rice crackers or baking soda biscuits, fresh fruit or cup of soup
- Rice pasta primavera, pickled beets, mixed green salad with vinaigrette, leftover breakfast rice pudding topped with berries

Snacks

- Rice cakes or crackers with ghee or unsweetened apple butter or coconut oil, raw carrot
- Guacamole on rice cakes
- Vegetables dipped into guacamole
- Baked apple
- Poached pear
- Bowl of soup and rice crackers
- Rice cakes or crackers spread with apple butter
- Fresh fruit
- Fresh vegetables: carrots, cucumbers, sweet peppers, etc.
- Mochi rice squares, plain or with apple butter or smashed berries
- Baked sweet potatoes

Recipes

One of the most challenging parts of an elimination diet is figuring out what you CAN eat for a meal. I remember my second and third weeks being the most difficult. I picked up a fantastic cookbook called Allergy Cooking With Ease by Nicolette M. Dumke aka the no wheat, milk, eggs, soy, yeast, sugar, grain, and gluten cookbook! This one has a bunch of safe ideas.

Another book I used for cost effective and delicious meals was Supermarket Healthy by Food Network's Melissa D'Arabian. I talk about both of these books a lot on my blog.

If you get stuck, there are tons of recipes on acleanfit.co, and they are all over Pinterest! Here are some recipes that I still enjoy from these two books.

Breakfast Rice Pudding

- Serves 4

1 cup uncooked short grain brown rice

1¼ cups coconut milk

1¼ cups water

½ tsp. salt

1 Tbsp. brown rice syrup

1 tsp. cinnamon

Combine water and coconut milk in heavy pot; bring to boil, adding rice and salt. Simmer, covered (do NOT stir) for about 45 minutes or more, until liquid is mostly absorbed and rice is soft . Remove from heat and allow to cool for 15 minutes. Stir in brown rice syrup and cinnamon.

Mochi Rice Waffles

- Serves 4

Purchase 1 package of cinnamon-apple Mochi and defrost. Cut into quarters. Slice each quarter across to form 2 thinner squares. Place one square into preheated waffle iron and cook until done. Top with your choice of fruit or Sautéed Apples (recipe below).

Rice Pancakes

- Makes approximately 14 (4-inch) pancakes

1 1/3 cups rice flour

½ cup millet flour

2 tsp. baking powder

½ tsp. baking soda

¼ tsp. salt

1 Tbsp. apple butter

1 Tbsp. ghee Egg Replacer to equal 2 eggs (Refer to recipe below.)

1½ cups rice milk

1½ Tbsp. apple cider vinegar

Mix the almond or rice milk with the vinegar and allow them to stand for 5 minutes until curdles form. Mix dry ingredients together and set aside. In large mixing bowl, beat apple butter, oil, egg, and milk. Add dry mixture and stir gently. Be careful not to over-mix. Serve with Sautéed Apples (refer to recipe below).

Sweet Potato Delight

- Serves 1-2

1 ripe banana

1 medium sweet potato, cooked

1 tsp. oil 1 Tbsp. fruit sweetener, molasses or brown rice syrup (optional)

Shake the pan often. Cut the banana in half lengthwise. Cut the cooked sweet potato into ½" pieces. Add the oil to the pan. Place the banana pieces, flat sides down, in the pan. Add the sweet potatoes. Cover and cook for 2 minutes. Uncover, and cook for 5 minutes, until everything is heated through and browned on one side. Add the sweetener before serving.

Lunch and Dinner

Oven Roasted Veggies

– number of servings depend on amount of veggies used

Use any combination of the following vegetables, unpeeled, washed, and cut into bite-sized pieces: eggplant, small red potatoes, red onion, yellow or green summer squash, mushrooms, asparagus. Toss with crushed garlic cloves, olive oil and sprinkle with rosemary, oregano, tarragon, and basil to taste. Spread in roasting pan in single layers and roast approximately 20-25 minutes at 400 degrees until veggies are tender and slightly brown, stirring occasionally. The amount of time needed depends on the size of the veggie. Salt and pepper to taste. Serve while warm, or use cold left overs in salad.

Mock Pesto

- Makes 1 cup

1 large ripe avocado

1 cup basil leaves

¼ tsp. lemon juice

1 garlic clove, minced or 1/8 tsp. garlic powder

¼ cup pine nuts

½ tsp. olive or flax oil

Cut the avocado in half and remove the pit. Scoop out the flesh and place it in a bowl of a food processor. Add the basil, lemon juice, garlic and pine nuts. Process for about 2 minutes – scrape the bowl as necessary. Transfer it to a small bowl and coat the surface with oil to prevent browning. Chill.

Rice Pasta Primavera

– Serves 4

2 cups uncooked rice pasta (noodles, spaghetti, elbows)

1 large whole chicken breast, cut into thin strips (optional)

Broccoli florets, chopped carrot, and/or other favorite veggie

lightly steamed 3-4 scallion chopped

2 cloves garlic, minced

1 Tbsp. olive oil (more if needed)

¼ cup fresh basil, finely chopped

¼ - ½ cup coconut milk

Cook rice pasta according to package directions. While pasta is cooking, heat oil in wok or heavy frying pan, and stir fry chicken strips or tofu chunks, garlic, scallions, and basil for about 5 minutes; add remaining vegetables and coconut milk and continue to cook until veggies are soft and glisten. Add more coconut milk as needed. Remove from heat and spoon over drained rice pasta and garnish with black olives and extra olive oil, if desired.

No Meat or Tomato Chili

The paprika and Vitamin C crystals add the color and tang to tomatoes to this vegetarian chili.

1/2c cold water or bean liquid

1 tsp. tapioca starch or arrowroot

1/16 to ⅛ tsp chili powder (or to taste)

1-½ - 2c cooked pinto or kidney beans

½ to ⅝ tsp tart-tasting unbuffered Vitamin C crystals, such as Vita Life brand

Combine with water or bean liquid and tapioca starch or arrowroot in a saucepan. Add the chili powder, paprika, and bring mixture to a boil, stirring it often. Add the beans, crushing a few of them against the side of the pan, and simmer the chili for a few minutes. Stir in the Vitamin C crystals. Serve the chili alone or over cooked rice, quinoa, or baked potatoes when you can!

Asparagus Soup

- Serves 4

1 lb. asparagus, trimmed

2 medium leeks or 4 large shallots

1 Tbsp. oil

2-3 cloves garlic, minced

2 cups water or chicken stock

1 tsp. dried dill weed

pinch nutmeg

Slice off the tips of the asparagus and reserve them. Cut the remaining stalks into 1" pieces. Slice the leeks in half lengthwise and wash under cold water to remove any sand. Slice into ¼" pieces. Sautée the leeks or shallots in the oil over medium heat until soft . Add the garlic and sliced asparagus stalks. Cook, stirring, another minute or two. Add the water or stock and dill. Simmer 10-12 minutes. Remove from heat, allow to cool 5-10 minutes. Puree half the volume at a time. Return to pan, add the reserved asparagus tips and simmer 3-5 minutes or until tips are just barely tender. Add nutmeg. If soup is too thick, thin with additional water or stock.

Basic Stock Recipe

In a stock pot: Put 2 pounds bones, skin, cartilage from poultry, fish, beef, lamb, shellfish. (If you use a whole chicken, cook for about an hour, then take meat off the bones. Toss bones and connective tissue back into the pot. Leave the meat aside.) Cover with water (2-3 quarts) 1-2 Tbsp. of lemon juice or vinegar, 1-2 tsp salt, ½ tsp pepper, carrots, onions, celery, parsley, sage, rosemary, thyme, bay. Cook several hours (4-24) or in crock pot on low temp. Skim off scum/solids from top of soup after a couple of hours. Remove bones. Skim off fat. (Sometimes it's easiest to refrigerate and then skim off fat.) Either strain and use as broth, or begin adding vegetables, grains, etc., to make a soup. Can be used to cook grains or vegetables instead of water.

Salads and Vegetables

Cabbage Salad

- Serves 4-6

1 small to medium head red cabbage, thinly sliced (or use half red and half green cabbage)

8 sliced radishes, or 1 grated carrot

3 green apples, diced

1 stalk celery, chopped

dash garlic powder

2 Tbsp. olive oil

2 tsp. vinegar

1 tsp. lemon juice

Mix all ingredients in a bowl and allow to sit for an hour, stirring once or twice. Serve cold or at room temperature.

Fruity Spinach Salad

- Serves 6-8

1 lb. fresh spinach, washed, dried, torn into pieces

1 pint fresh organic strawberries or raspberries, washed

Dressing:

3 Tbsp pine nuts

2 scallions, chopped

½ cup olive or flax oil

¼ cup balsamic vinegar

Cut berries in half and arrange over spinach in serving bowl. Combine dressing ingredients in blender or food processor and process until smooth. Just before serving, pour over salad and toss. Garnish with nuts.

Guacamole

- Makes 1 ½ - 2 cups

2-3 ripe avocados

¼ cup chopped onions

¼ tsp. vitamin C crystals

1 Tbsp. water

1 small clove garlic, chopped

Cut the avocados in half, remove the pits, then scoop the flesh into a blender or food processor. Add the onions, vitamin C crystals, water, and garlic. Process until smooth. Transfer to a small bowl. Cover and chill. Use within 2-3 days. To prevent darkening, coat top with a thin layer of oil. For a chunky version, mash the avocado with a fork and finely chop onions and garlic.

Pickled Beets

- Serves 4-6

4 beets, cooked and skinned

¼ cup water

1 Tbsp. brown rice syrup or fruit sweetener

¼ cup rice vinegar

¼ tsp. ground cinnamon pinch each of cloves and allspice

Combine the water, sweetener, vinegar, cinnamon, cloves and allspice in a medium saucepan. Simmer for 2 minutes. Stir in the beets, and heat through. Serve hot or warm.

Quinoa Salad

- Serves 8-10

1 ½ cups quinoa, rinsed several times

3 cups water, or chicken broth or vegetable broth (or a combination)

1 cup fresh or frozen peas (frozen baby peas should be just defrosted)

Chopped veggies, raw or lightly steamed (broccoli, asparagus, green beans, etc)

½ cup chopped red onion

1 pint cherry tomatoes (optional)

½ cup chopped black olives (optional)

1/3 cup olive oil

2 Tbsp. balsamic vinegar or lemon juice

1 or 2 crushed garlic cloves

2-4 Tbsp. fresh dill, chopped (or 1 Tbsp. dried dill)

2 Tbsp. chopped fresh parsley salt and pepper to taste

Rinse quinoa well (quinoa tastes bitter if not well rinsed). Bring 3 cups water or broth to a boil. Add rinsed quinoa and bring back to boil. Simmer uncovered for about 15 minutes until liquid is well absorbed. Transfer to large bowl with a small amount of olive oil to prevent sticking, and allow to cool. Meantime, mix together remaining oil, vinegar or lemon juice, parsley, and garlic in a small bowl. Add veggies to quinoa and toss well with dressing mixture, dill, salt and pepper. Chill before serving.

Vinaigrette Dressing

- 6 servings (approximately)

Note: ingredient amounts in this recipe are approximate; use more or less of certain ingredients to adapt recipe to your personal taste.

½ cup extra-virgin

Olive oil

3 Tbsp. balsamic vinegar (preferred because it has the richest flavor)

2-3 Tbsp. water

1 tsp. dry mustard

1-3 cloves fresh garlic (whole pieces for flavor or crushed for stronger taste)

Salt and pepper to taste

Oregano, basil, parsley, tarragon or any herbs of your choice, fresh or dried

Place vinegar, water and mustard in a tightly capped jar, and shake well to thoroughly dissolve mustard. Add oil and remaining ingredients and shake well again. Store refrigerated and shake well before using. Dressing will harden when cold; allow 5-10 minutes to re-liquify.

Grains/Breads

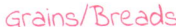

Basic Kasha

Serves 4-5

1 cup buckwheat groats

2 cups water, chicken or vegetable broth

Roast the dry buckwheat groats over medium heat in a dry skillet, stirring until the grains begin to smell toasty, about 2 minutes. Add the water or broth, cover and simmer for 20-30 minutes, until kasha is tender but not mushy. Pour off any excess liquid. Optional: add onion, garlic and herbs to the dish.

Baking Powder Biscuits

- Makes 12

1½ cups brown rice flour

½ cup tapioca flour

4 tsp. baking powder

1/8 tsp. salt

3 Tbsp. ghee

1 cup applesauce, unsweetened

Preheat oven to 425 degrees. In a medium-large mixing bowl, stir together dry ingredients. Sprinkle oil on top and mix well with a pastry blender or fork, until consistency is crumbly. Mix in applesauce and stir until blended. Spoon heaping tablespoonfuls onto ungreased cookie sheet. With spoon, lightly shape into biscuit. Bake 15-18 minutes until slightly browned. Serve warm for best flavor, but may be lightly reheated in a microwave.

Green Rice

- Serves 4

1 cup brown basmati rice

2 cups water

¼ to½ tsp salt

1 bunch parsley

1 clove garlic

1½ Tbsp. lemon juice

1½ Tbsp. olive oil

½ cucumber, diced

Pepper to taste

Bring water to a boil, add rice and salt, stir and simmer, covered, for 45 minutes. Remove from heat and let sit for another 10 minutes; then remove cover and allow to cool. While rice is cooking, blend almonds, parsley, garlic, and oil in a food processor. When rice is cool, stir with nut mixture and add pepper to taste. Garnish with cucumber if desired.

Meal in a Muffin

– Makes 12

1 medium carrot, grated

1 large apple, grated

¼ cup ghee

¼ cup unsweetened applesauce

Egg Replacement to equal 2 eggs

1/3 cup rice syrup, molasses, or agave (or mixture of those sweeteners)

2 tsp. vanilla

¼ cup millet flour

½ cup brown rice flour

¼ tsp. cinnamon

½ tsp. baking powder

¼ tsp. ginger

1/8 tsp. nutmeg

¼ cup shredded unsweetened coconut

½ cup dates

Preheat oven to 375 degrees. Mix together all wet ingredients and set aside. In a separate bowl, mix dry ingredients then mix both together. Lightly coat muffin tins with oil spray. Fill 3/4 full and bake 15-20 minutes or until toothpick comes out clean. Allow to cool on a rack.

Yellow Rice

2 cups chicken stock
1 small onion, finely chopped
2 tsp. olive oil
1 clove garlic, minced
½ tsp. turmeric
1 cup uncooked long-grain brown rice

In a 2-quart saucepan over low heat, sauté onions in oil until tender, about 5 minutes. Add the garlic and sauté 1 minute. Stir in turmeric, then rice. Add stock. Bring to a boil, cover and simmer 45 minutes over low heat, or until rice is tender and all liquid is absorbed. Do not stir. Spoon beans over rice.

Fruit

Baked Apple

- Serves 6

1/3 cup golden raisins

2 Tbsp. apple juice

6 cooking apples, cored

1½ cups water

¼ cup frozen unsweetened apple juice concentrate

2 tsp. pure vanilla extract

1 tsp. cinnamon

1 tsp. arrowroot

Remove peel from top third of each apple and arrange in a small baking dish. In a medium saucepan, combine other ingredients and bring to a boil, stirring frequently. Reduce heat and simmer 2-3 minutes, until slightly thickened. Distribute raisins, filling centers of each apple. Pour sauce over apples and bake, uncovered, at 350 degrees for 1 to 1 1/2 hours. Baste occasionally and remove from oven when apples are pierced easily with a fork. Spoon juice over apples and serve warm.

Poached Pears

– Serves 6

6 pears

2-inch stick cinnamon or 1 tsp. cinnamon

1 t. cardamom

2 c. apple juice or apple cranberry juice

Peel pears or leave whole. Place in covered casserole in oven or soup pot on stove. Cook until soft –30-60 minutes depending on the ripeness of the pears.

Sautéed Apples

- Serves 2

2 apples, washed

½ Tbsp. olive oil or ghee

2 tsp. cinnamon

2-3 Tbsp. apple juice

Thinly slice apples and sauté in oil until softened. Add cinnamon and apple juice and simmer, stirring, uncovered for a few more minutes.

Corn-Free Baking Powder

2 tsp. cream of tartar

2 tsp. arrowroot

1 tsp. baking soda

Sift together to mix well. Store in an airtight container. Make small batches.

Egg Replacer

- equals one egg

1/3 cup water

1 Tbsp.whole or ground flaxseed

Place the water and flaxseed together and allow to gel for about 5 minutes. This mixture will bind patties, meat loaves, cookies and cakes as well as eggs do, but it will not leaven like eggs for souffles or sponge cakes. Increase amounts accordingly for additional egg replacement.

Nutty Mayo
- Makes 1¼ cups. (Keeps well for 3 weeks)
½ cup pine nuts
¾ cup water
3 Tbsp. vinegar
2 Tbsp. oil
1 Tbsp. arrowroot
1 Tbsp. brown rice syrup
1 Tbsp. minced parsley
1 Tbsp. snipped chives
1½ tsp. dry mustard

Grind the pine nuts to a fi ne powder in a blender. Add the water, blend 1 minute to make sure the pine nuts are fully ground. Add the vinegar, oil, arrowroot, sweetener, and seasonings. Blend until very smooth. Pour into a saucepan and cook a few minutes, until thick. Allow to cool.

MEGA LOVE ON YOUR JOURNEY

Congratulations to you on the beginning of your newest adventure! Positive vibes are heading in your direction, simply because you took initiative. Remind yourself *daily* how important your wellbeing is, and to be patient while you work. I also want you to remember that change takes a challenge! Now you have the tools and the courage to take with you to discover the root of your challenge. I'm rooting for you!

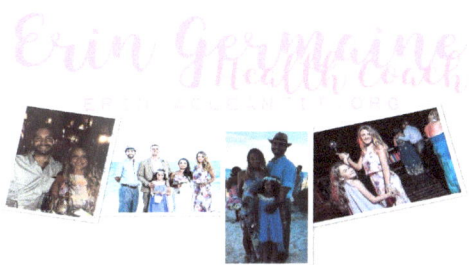

www.ingramcontent.com/pod-product-compliance
Lightning Source LLC
Chambersburg PA
CBHW050831290526
45792CB00001B/352